# THE
# MEDITERRANEAN ANTI-AGING SECRET

**TERRY LEMEROND**

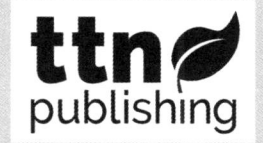

ttn publishing

The purpose of this book is to educate. It is not intended to serve as a replacement for professional medical advice. Any use of the information in this book is at the reader's discretion. This book is sold with the understanding that neither the publisher nor the authors have any liability or responsibility for any injury caused or alleged to be caused directly or indirectly by the information contained in this book. While every effort has been made to ensure its accuracy, the book's contents should not be construed as medical advice. To obtain medical advice on your individual health needs, please consult a qualified health care practitioner.

Copyright © 2023 TTN Publishing, LLC, Green Bay, WI

All rights reserved. Except as permitted under the United States Copyright Act of 1976, no part of this publication in any format, electronic or physical, may be reproduced or distributed in any form or by any means, or stored in a database or retrieval system without the prior written permission of the publisher.

Library of Congress Cataloging-in-Publication Data is on file with the Library of Congress.

ISBN: 978-1-952507-38-0

Editor: Kathleen Barnes • www.takechargebooks.com
Interior design: Gary A. Rosenberg • www.thebookcouple.com

Printed in the United States of America

10   9   8   7   6   5   4   3   2   1

# Contents

Chapter 1. A Gift from Mount Olympus ............... 1

Chapter 2. What Gives GMT Its Kick? ................. 7

Chapter 3. What Is Alzheimer's Disease? ............. 13

Chapter 4. How GMT Treats and Even
Reverses Alzheimer's Disease ............ 21

Chapter 5. GMT and Brain Function ................... 27

Chapter 6. GMT's Other Benefits ...................... 35

Chapter 7. Add in Bacopa ............................. 41

Chapter 8. The Right Combo ........................... 47

Chapter 9. Doc to Doc—
For Healthcare Professionals ............... 51

*References* ............................................. 57

*Index* .................................................. 59

*About the Author* ..................................... 63

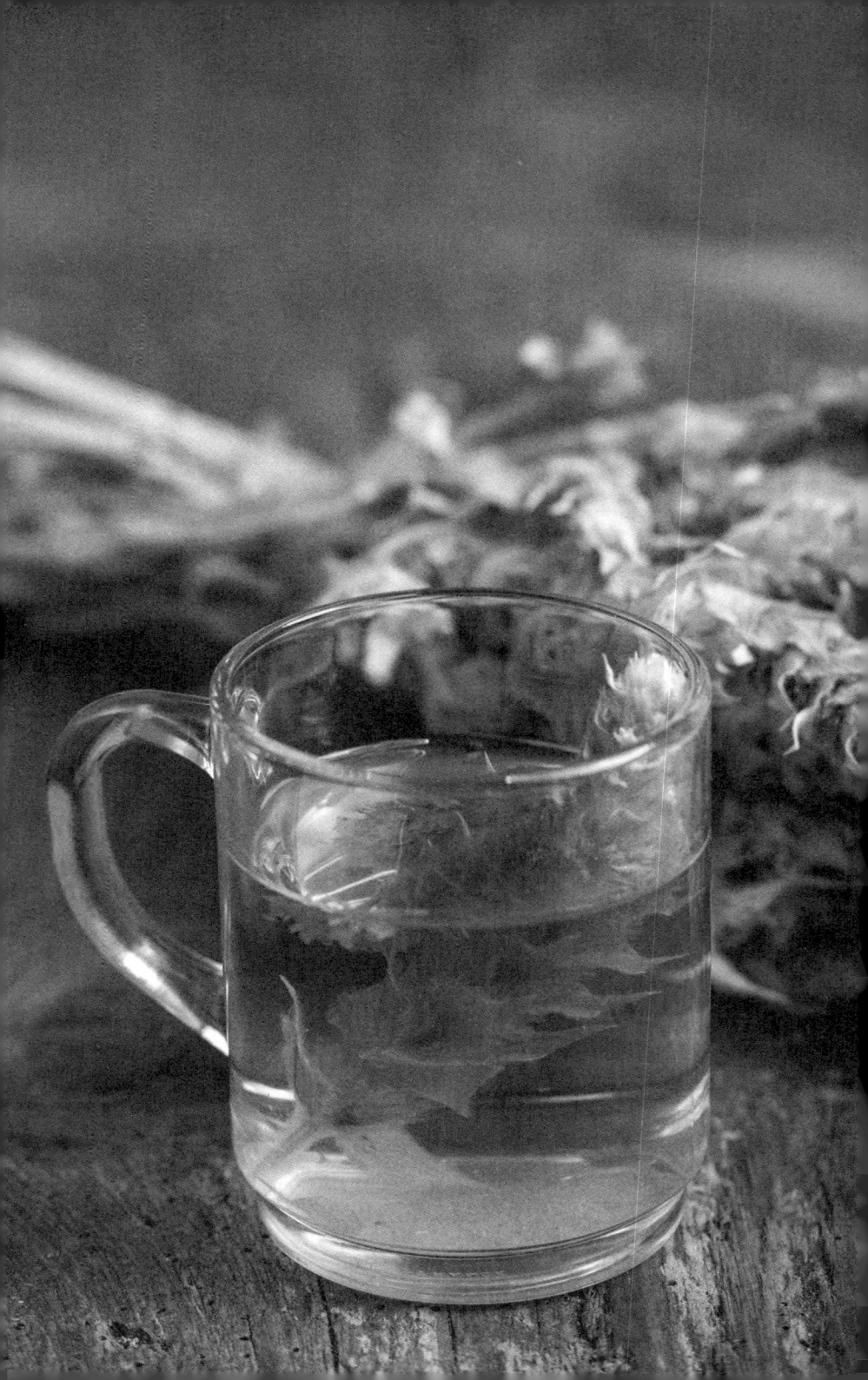

## CHAPTER 1

# A Gift from Mount Olympus

Mount Olympus is the legendary home of the Greek gods. It's the mythological home of the most revered symbols of the ancient Greek religion as well as a physical symbol, it's one of Europe's highest peaks soaring more than 9,500 feet above the serene Aegean Sea.

The sacred mountain is a high, dry chaparral with a wealth of biodiversity.

How could there be a better birthplace for one of Mother Nature's greatest healing gifts?

I'm talking about Greek Mountain Tea *(Sideritis scardica: translation "he who is made of iron"),* frequently called "Olympos" tea by Greeks and their Mediterranean neighbors. Also called "ironwort" or "shepherd's tea," Greek Mountain Tea (GMT) grows wild at altitudes above 3,200 feet.

It's a survivor, growing wild and thriving on poor soil and limited amounts of water. Most Greek Mountain Tea is wild grown, harvested by local farmers and minimally processed at those same high altitudes.

Its popularity is well-deserved. In ancient times, Greek shepherds began to harvest GMT to help them stay healthy, warm and mentally alert. Hippocrates, the father of modern medicine, lauded GMT's benefits for immune dysfunction and respiratory illnesses. Greeks still use the tea today to combat winter colds and flu.

They also used GMT for wound healing, especially wounds caused by iron weapons, hence the nickname "ironwort." Today's research confirms that GMT's antimicrobial qualities help prevent wounds from becoming infected.

## Vast healing power

In modern times, GMT has been widely acclaimed for its vast healing power. Modern scientific research confirms GMT can:

▲ Combat Alzheimer's disease

▲ Lower blood pressure, reducing the risk of heart attacks and strokes

▲ Improve digestive health

▲ Increase bone density

▲ Enhance immune function and prevent colds and flu

▲ Reduce anxiety and depression

▲ Reduce insulin resistance

▲ Promote weight loss

▲ Relieve joint pain

The most exciting for me is GMT's effectiveness against Alzheimer's disease and dementia, confirmed through several well-researched published studies.

Alzheimers disease and dementia are the subjects of this book, so these findings will be addressed in great detail.

Let me just say for now that conventional medicine has been unable to find any long-term solution to Alzheimer's, the heartrending disease sometimes called The Long Goodbye.

## How does it work?

GMT's considerable healing properties are attributed to aromatic essential oils and antioxidant-rich polyphenols and flavonoids.

### What's an antioxidant and why is it important?

While we need to breathe oxygen to stay alive, oxygen in our cells works just as destructively as it does on that plain apple. When a cut apple is exposed to air, it turns brown. This is a process called oxidation. A similar process happens in human cells. Lifestyle choices and exposure to environmental toxins over a lifetime causes cells to "brown," like on an apple. Actually, the correct terminology is free radical oxygen molecules. These molecules collect and accumulate in your cells. They trigger chronic inflammation, opening the door to cell aging and genetic deterioration, as well as to the diseases of aging, including cancer, heart disease, diabetes and yes, dementia and Alzheimer's.

### What are antioxidants, you might ask?

Harvard scientists give us a simple explanation: "Antioxidants neutralize free radicals by giving up some of their own electrons. In making this sacrifice, they act as a natural "off" switch for the free radicals. This helps break a chain reaction that can affect other molecules in the cell and other cells in the body."

At least 90% of all of our modern-day diseases are caused by oxidative stress and inflammation.

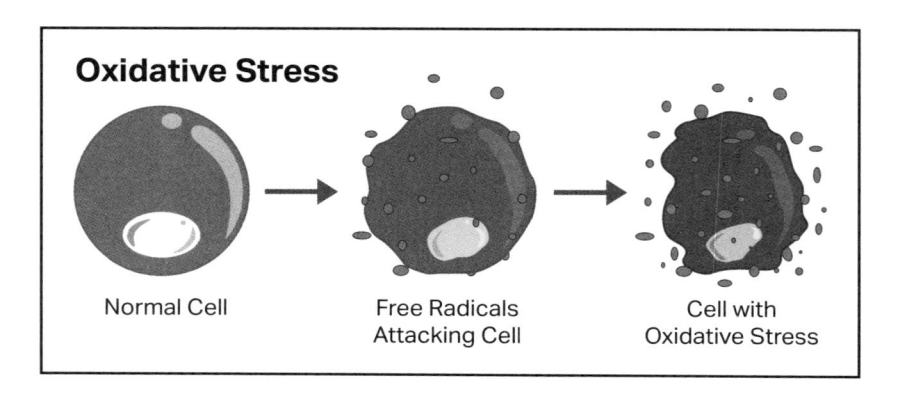

**Oxidative Stress**

Normal Cell → Free Radicals Attacking Cell → Cell with Oxidative Stress

Science has also shown us that most chronic disease is caused by lifestyle choices and environmental influences. Simple dietary and exercise choices can have a profoundly positive effect on your health.

This means choosing an antioxidant-rich diet that includes an abundance of colorful fruits and vegetables, spices, and healing tea, like GMT.

Greek Mountain Tea has at least the antioxidant content as green tea, without the caffeine that troubles some people, so you can take it anytime through the day and evening.

Those antioxidants come from a nutrient group called polyphenols. Science has shown us over and over again that a diet rich in polyphenols derived mainly from fruits, vegetables, and beverages such as tea, coffee, olive oil or wine is valued in the prevention of premature aging, cardiovascular disease and even cancer.

We can confidently add Greek Mountain Tea to that list.

Plus, GMT has strong anti-inflammatory benefits. We know that inflammation contributes to oxidative stress and is an underlying cause of all of the diseases mentioned in the paragraphs above.

I'll go into the details in depth in the coming chapters, but I can say without any doubt right now that Greek Mountain Tea should be a part of the daily regimen of anyone who has been diagnosed with Alzheimer's disease or dementia, or even any type of cognitive decline.

I'll go a step farther and say that I think anyone over 60 should consider taking GMT daily. If you choose to drink 2–3 cups of organic tea daily, you'll be delighted with its slightly sweet flowery taste.

While the tea is pleasant, it does require time to prepare. Now, for the first time, GMT is available in capsule form, offering all of the benefits of the healing tea without the hassle of preparation. Since I travel a lot, I'm really happy to be able to pack a bottle of capsules in my carry-on and know how easy it is to take a capsule or two a day and have the peace of mind that I'm protecting myself from the diseases of aging.

Read on. I'm sure you'll agree with me that GMT offers answers to questions that conventional medicine hasn't been able to address.

## WHAT YOU NEED TO KNOW...

Greek Mountain Tea (GMT) has been used by Greeks and the people of the Mediterranean region for millennia for a wide variety of healing purposes.

Traditionally, GMT was used as:

- ▲ A tonic to prevent colds and flu
- ▲ An antiseptic to prevent wounds from becoming infected
- ▲ An antidepressant

Now, modern science confirms GMT's effectiveness as it was used in ancient times, plus it can:

- ▲ Combat Alzheimer's disease and cognitive dysfunction
- ▲ Lower blood pressure, reducing the risk of heart attacks and strokes
- ▲ Improve digestive health
- ▲ Increase bone density
- ▲ Reduce insulin resistance
- ▲ Promote weight loss
- ▲ Relieve joint pain

## CHAPTER 2
# What Gives GMT Its Kick?

Greek Mountain Tea looks and smells a bit like sage and it thrives in the same challenging hot and dry growing conditions. Perhaps it's that hardy nature that helps GMT create the host of protective compounds that make it such a valuable healing plant.

Tea brewed from the leaves, stems and flowers of the *Sideritis scardica* plant or a simple extract in a capsule offers impressive benefits to the human body.

## Polyphenols

At the top of the list is a long list of tongue-twisting polyphenols. I'll add them at the end of this section for my scientifically-inclined readers. It's important to know that polyphenols are an essential part of the wealth of nutrients provided for use by Mother Nature.

Maybe you haven't heard of the word "polyphenol" before. It's a blanket term for any of the 8,000 super healthy nutrients found in fruits, vegetables, herbs and bee products.

Maybe words like flavonoids, catechins, anthocyanins, lignans, quercetin, curcuminoids, resveratrol, ellagic acid and phenolic acids are a bit daunting. They're all polyphenols, too.

I'm sure that you've all heard of caffeine, another important polyphenol.

These are all in the family of polyphenols that give fruits, vegetables, flowering herbs (like GMT) and spices their glowing colors and aromas and serve as natural antibiotics, insecticides and cellular protectors for the plant world.

Not surprisingly, the polyphenols are also potent and natural protectors of human health. Since the human body cannot synthesize or store polyphenols, we rely on continuous replenishment by daily diet.

Polyphenols are so important because of their supercharged antioxidant and anti-inflammatory properties.

## Antioxidant wealth

In Chapter 1, we looked a little bit at free radical oxygen molecules and the importance of antioxidants to counter the cellular deterioration that is an underlying cause of most chronic diseases.

Inflammation and free radical damage go hand-in-hand. It's hard to say which comes first, the chicken or the egg, the free radical or the inflammation, but one almost always accompanies the other resulting in cellular damage, escalated aging process and disease.

Antioxidants are rated on a scale called ORAC according to their capacity to neutralize free radical oxygen molecules. In fact, GMT has a higher antioxidant value per serving than blueberries and blackberries, considered to be among the most potent antioxidant foods.

Since polyphenols are the most important antioxidants, it's important to know that GMT has a similar polyphenol level to apples and red raspberries.

## ORAC Values

**Greek Mountain Tea:** 6,900 to 7,400 umol per serving

**Blueberries:** 6,552 umol per serving

**Blackberries:** 5,347 umol per serving

GMT's total content of bioflavonoids, which are an important subcategory of polyphenols, is twice what you'd get in a cup of chamomile tea.

Polish researchers who delved deeply into the composition of GMT also found "appreciable quantities" of other healthy plant nutrients, including apigenin, quercetin, kaempherol, and caffeic and chlorogenic acids.

For those of you who like to know the science, here's the promised list of unique compounds that comprise about 90% of the polyphenols in GMT and are the source of its antioxidant, anti-inflammatory and brain protective benefits:

- ▲ Phenylethanoid glycosides
- ▲ Flavonoid acetyl glycosides (mainly apigenin, luteolin, isoscutellarein and hypolaetin derivatives)
- ▲ Hydroxycinnamic acid derivatives, mainly ferulic acid and caffeic acid
- ▲ Echinacoside
- ▲ Lavandulifoloside
- ▲ Verbascoside
- ▲ ForsythosideA
- ▲ Isoverbascoside
- ▲ Samioside
- ▲ Allysonoside
- ▲ Leucoseptoside
- ▲ A broad range of acetyl glycosides

## Minerals

GMT is also a rich source of health-promoting minerals. The pivotal Polish research confirms that GMT is a healthy source of:

- Potassium
- Magnesium
- Iron
- Phosphorus
- Sodium
- Copper
- Calcium
- Manganese
- Zinc

Minerals are vital to almost every function of the human body. They:

- Convert food into energy
- Build proteins
- Repair cell damage
- Promote optimal brain function
- Boost heart health
- Strengthen teeth and bones
- Boost energy levels
- Regulate blood sugar levels
- Maintain muscle health
- Trigger immunity
- Create healthy DNA and exact replication of cells
- Manufacture red blood cells
- Heal damaged tissue
- Support the nervous system
- Balance thyroid function
- Manufacture hormones and digestive enzymes
- Maintain electrolyte balance, keep fluids stable

From these lists, it's easy to see that the minerals found in GMT are a valuable addition to the antioxidant and anti-inflammatory benefits we've already mentioned.

## There's more . . .

The ancient Greeks who used GMT for wound healing and to prevent colds and flu (and many modern Greek and Mediterranean people still do) are now confirmed by modern science. The antimicrobial properties of GMT show that monoterpenes such as α-pinene, β-pinene, and carvacrol have proven antimicrobial properties including killing infectious bacteria, antibacterial, and killing harmful fungi.

Add in the boosting power of essential oils like free radical fighting pinene and food-poisoning busting carvacrol and it all adds up to some profound healing power.

I don't think I need to pursue these lines any further to convince you that the health benefits of Greek Mountain Tea are impressive, important and essential to improving your health.

## WHAT YOU NEED TO KNOW . . .

Greek Mountain Tea (GMT) contains a wealth of health benefits that protect against most chronic diseases associated with aging.

GMT is a rich source of polyphenols, antioxidant and anti-inflammatory nutrient molecules, vital minerals, and health-promoting essential oils.

Among the many benefits of GMT are protection against:

▲ Alzheimer's disease

▲ ADHD and other brain dysfunction

▲ Cardiovascular disease

▲ Type 2 diabetes

▲ Several forms of cancer

▲ Gastrointestinal distress

▲ Anxiety and depression

# CHAPTER 3

# What Is Alzheimer's Disease?

In 1995, Former President Ronald Reagan, then 83 years old, wrote a letter to the public announcing he was afflicted with Alzheimer's disease.

In the ensuing nine years until his death, his family and in some ways, the public, engaged with Reagan in what his daughter, Patti Davis, called "the Long Goodbye" in her 2005 book, a year after his death.

This disease, that Davis describes saying goodbye to her father in stages as Alzheimer's stole what is most precious—a person's memory. "Alzheimer's," she writes, "snips away at the threads, a slow unraveling, a steady retreat; as a witness all you can do is watch, cry, and whisper a soft stream of goodbyes."

The Reagans brought into the public eye the agony of the disease that so many of us have endured. In fact, today, at least 5.8 million Americans (and their families) are living with the disease.

I bring in their families because perhaps the only merciful part of Alzheimer's disease is that the person suffering from the disease is rarely aware of the progression from moderate to severe memory loss and dementia.

The family is painfully aware. The emotional and financial effects of Alzheimer's are devastating. It can rip families apart as caregiving requirements and decisions when to enter institutionalized care take their toll.

## What is Alzheimer's?

Alzheimer's disease (AD) is a brain disorder that slowly destroys memory and thinking skills and, eventually, the ability to carry out the simplest tasks, according to the National Institute on Aging.

Alzheimer's disease is a "progressive" brain disease characterized by changes in the brain that can affect a person's ability to remember and think and, eventually, to live independently. "Progressive" is a euphemism for irreversible, deteriorating and terminal. In the end stage of AD, the body literally forgets how to swallow or breathe or digest food.

The average person lives eight years after a diagnosis with AD.

But read on, my friends. As dire as the diagnosis has been in the past, new research on Greek Mountain Tea may be a game changer.

## Causes

Scientists don't yet fully understand what causes AD, but they speculate it is a combination of age-related changes in the brain along with genetic, environmental and lifestyle factors.

The importance of any one of these factors in increasing or decreasing the risk of AD are uniquely individual.

One thing I firmly believe applies to everyone: Use it or

lose it. That means that we should all challenge our brains as much as possible. Read novels and nonfiction. Discuss current events. Take a ballroom dance class where you have to memorize steps. Learn a foreign language. Go for a walk with a friend. Do crossword puzzles or, if you're really good at them, do math puzzles.

Simply exercise your brain like you'd exercise the rest of your body. I'm of a certain age myself and I know I have to work at brain health the older I get.

Until now, modern science has validated several prescription drugs that can slow the progression of AD, but some have serious and sometimes lethal side effects. Preventives and cures have been elusive.

Botanicals have been in traditional use for millennia. Some, like GMT, are now validated for effectiveness without side effects.

## What happens in the brains of people diagnosed with Alzheimer's?

CT scans can show brain shrinkage, a key to diagnose the disease, but CT scans can't tell the difference between AD and other forms of dementia that may be caused by a lack of blood flow to the brain often caused by a stroke, toxic exposures, vitamin deficiencies and Parkinson's disease.

People with AD typically have clumps of protein called beta amyloid plaques that form between the nerve cells in the brain. They develop primarily in the areas of the brain that govern memory and cognitive function.

Think of brain function likes an electrical system. Brain cells called neurons that have long finger-like extensions called dendrites that reach out to other neurons to create an information pathway. Brain signals literally travel from neuron to neuron through those dendrite connections. Amyloid plaques and thread-like accumulations of protein called tau tangles block the neural information system.

As you might guess from the first two chapters of this book, inflammation plays a major role in this deterioration by destroying the brain's natural filtration and waste destroying system.

## Stages

There are five recognized stages of AD.

1. Preclinical disease that would only be determined in research settings and may be present for years before the individual or family recognize its onset.

2. Mild cognitive impairment (MCI) with mild changes in memory and thinking skills. These are probably not severe enough to affect work or relationships.

3. Mild dementia that includes memory loss of recent events, difficulty with problem solving or judgment-related tasks.

4. Personality changes including becoming withdrawn or inexplicably angry or irritable.

5. Deepening confusion, increasingly poor judgment, deepening memory loss like forgetting their address, needing help with daily tasks like toileting and hygiene, and significant personality changes and delusions.

Pneumonia is a common cause of death in late-stage Alzheimer's patients because loss of the ability to swallow allows food or beverages to enter the lungs, where an infection can begin. Dehydration, malnutrition, falls and other types of infections are other common causes of death.

## An Alzheimer's diagnosis

Until about 20 years ago, an autopsy was the only way to definitively diagnose AD. Thankfully, science has made major advances in these two decades.

We can only hope that a cure will be found in the coming years.

Diagnosing AD is still not a precise science. Today, getting a definitive diagnosis is a multi-step process.

▲ The first step toward a diagnosis may be a simple word recall test to determine how good your short-term memory is.

▲ Other tests may measure problem solving abilities, attention, counting and language skills.

▲ Blood, urine and other standard medical tests might help rule out other medical issues that could cause memory loss.

▲ A psychiatric evaluation may be conducted to determine if depression, anxiety or other mental health challenges are causing the condition.

▲ A spinal tap may be conducted to measure proteins associated with AD and other types of dementia.

▲ Finally, brain scans including CT, MRI and PET may be conducted, largely to rule out other medical issues.

## ARCD or AD?

No doubt you've heard someone joke about having a "senior moment." Maybe you've even had some yourself.

It's normal to have such moments, even if you're 30! Science calls it age-related cognitive decline (ARCD) and confirms it is quite normal and common to forget where you left your car keys—or even where you parked your car—or why you walked into a room or even forgot your best friend's name.

Such memory lapses might be a cause for concern or not. As the rest of the body declines with age, so does the brain. Missing the thread of a conversation or losing your train of thought, or even forgetting a dentist appointment are all a part of life over 60.

Serious mental lapses that have a deep effect on your way of life or your ability to function in your daily life and your work life are causes for concern.

If you or your family members are concerned, seek medical advice.

## If you or someone you love has been diagnosed with AD

Conventional healthcare practitioners will encourage you to take one of the drugs that slows the progression. But they slow the progression with a cost. They may cause brain swelling, seizures, confusion, delirium and death.

Read on. There's a better and safer way.

## WHAT YOU NEED TO KNOW...

▲ Short-term memory loss is one of the first signs of Alzheimer's disease (AD), a progressive disease that begins with memory loss and ends in death several years later.

▲ Diagnosis is complex and usually begins with word recall, problem solving and other psychological tests followed by blood tests, brain scans and even spinal taps to determine if the problems are caused by AD.

▲ Several drugs have been approved to slow the progression of the disease, but they carry potentially severe side effects.

▲ There is no cure for AD.

CHAPTER 4

# How GMT Treats and Even Reverses Alzheimer's Disease

Greek Mountain Tea (GMT) has come onto the radar screens of modern-day researchers for its ability to prevent and/or dissipate the classic signs of Alzheimer's disease (AD), relieve outside factors that increase AD symptoms and perhaps even reverse the course of the disease.

They've been well-rewarded for their efforts.

A little background: Over the past decades, we've learned that depression, anxiety and impaired mental function are all connected, especially in the elderly. It's nearly impossible to separate the three. Researchers have also learned that treating one of those three elements can help improve the other two.

So, for example, if a person is both depressed and anxious (this is common), treating one or both of those conditions may also help improve cognitive function. If we can find a way to relieve depression, we can perhaps also relieve the symptoms of anxiety and improve cognitive function.

Research confirms that GMT works in several different ways.

**It acts as a triple monoamine reuptake inhibitor and increases blood flow in the brain.** I like to give you the scientific terminology for these things, but this is just a complicated way of saying it works as an antidepressant. In fact, this new category of antidepressants is at the forefront of expanded ways to treat depression and anxiety.

Increased blood flow to the brain, like increased blood flow to any organ, improves its function.

A 2018 British clinical trial of healthy older adults confirms both functions of GMT.

They found that in just 28 days, study subjects given standardized tests for depression, anxiety and cognitive function significantly reduced all three.

Compared to a group of patients given placebos and another group given *Ginkgo biloba*, a botanical often considered helpful in improving these symptoms, the group that received 950 mg of GMT:

▲ Had significantly better blood flow to the brain, possibly the underlying reason for the following improvements.

▲ Improved blood flow to the brain's prefrontal cortex, the part of the brain associated with cognitive behavior, personality expression, decision making and appropriate social behavior, all of which can be absent in people with AD.

▲ Improved their ability to remain focused and access working memory.

▲ Reduced their anxiety.

▲ Improved mood.

▲ Improved their ability to recognize pictures.

▲ Improved their ability to process information.

▲ Increased reaction speed.

▲ Improved overall cognitive performance.

▲ Improved transport of blood oxygen from the lungs to all other body tissues, including the brain.

Those British researchers, who also examined previous studies of GMT confirm its ability to ease anxiety and cognitive dysfunction as well as affirming that treating one element of the disease triad results in improvement of the others.

Let's take a look at some other important studies on GMT, polyphenols and brain health:

▲ **Enhance memory and learning abilities in animals with Alzheimer's:** A joint German-Norwegian study published in 2016 confirmed highly enhanced cognitive function in elderly lab animals, implying that GMT "might be a potent, well-tolerated option for treating symptoms of cognitive impairment in the elderly…"

▲ **Stop the formation of beta amyloid plaques:** This German animal study confirmed GMT's ability to slow or stop the formation of beta amyloid plaques, which you'll remember from Chapter 3 is one of the major characteristics of AD. The researchers concluded that further study is warranted to confirm the exact mechanism of action and the dosage necessary to treat and prevent clumping beta amyloid plaque.

▲ **Polyphenols improve cognitive function and protect the aging brain:** This German study looked at the benefits of polyphenol supplements in general. More than 4,000 studies on healthy elderly human subjects concluded that a dosage of at least 500 mg of various polyphenols was able to cross the blood-brain barrier, something few botanicals or pharmaceuticals can do, and significantly improve information processing speed, executive function and neuron function, while they reduce inflammation and free radical oxygen damage in the brain.

▲ **Overcome the limitations of chronic stress to improve cognitive performance:** This German study confirmed that GMT combined with vitamins B1, B6 and B12 helped human subjects overcome the stress caused by trying to concentrate during a test to improve their working memory, executive function, flexibility and stress behavior, while contending with a challenging noisy background atmosphere.

## Finally . . .

If you or someone you love has Alzheimer's in your family (there is a genetic component), I highly recommend that you consider adding GMT to your health regimen.

## WHAT YOU NEED TO KNOW . . .

Greek Mountain Tea is research-proven to prevent and treat Alzheimer's disease in several ways:

▲ It improves blood flow to the section of the brain that governs memory and other key functions that deteriorate in AD.

▲ It slows or stops the formation of beta amyloid plaque that is a major indicator of the disease.

▲ It improves communication along the network of brain cells.

▲ It combats depression and anxiety, which often go hand-in-hand with Alzheimer's.

▲ It improves memory, executive function, information processing speed and thinking effectiveness during stress.

▲ It reduces inflammation and free radical oxygen damage to the brain.

▲ Combined with *Bacopa monnieri,* GMT has been shown to improve working memory, focus and ability to concentrate during repetitive tasks.

# CHAPTER 5

# GMT and Brain Function

While the new science around Greek Mountain Tea (GMT) and Alzheimer's is a tremendously exciting development, there's more.

GMT works by a wide range of pathways to improve brain health by:

- ▲ Improving test scores
- ▲ Improving focus and concentration
- ▲ Relieving ADHD
- ▲ Creating a sense of calm alertness
- ▲ Improving scores on high-pressure, rapid-fire visual challenges
- ▲ Relieving stress and anxiety

## Blood-brain barrier

"The brain is precious, and evolution has gone to great lengths to protect it from damage," says the Queensland (Australia) Brain Institute.

GMT is one of the rare substances that can cross the blood-brain barrier (BBB), an exceptionally tight-knit network of blood vessels that activates the body's immune system to protect the brain from harm. I think of it as the security checkpoint between the brain and the rest of the body.

Only water, certain gases like oxygen, amino acids (protein molecules) and fat-soluble substances can easily pass from the blood into the brain. Other essential nutrients like glucose (blood sugar) enter the brain indirectly by "hitchhiking" on specific proteins.

The BBB prevents bacteria, fungi, viruses, parasites and other toxins that may be circulating in the bloodstream from entering the brain and causing infections that can be fatal. It's one of Mother Nature's most powerful ways of protecting us from serious illness and even death from infections like meningitis, HIV, some pneumonia-causing bacteria, *Streptococcus* and *E. coli* pathogens that can be present in your bloodstream.

Certain chronic diseases can weaken the BBB making it more easily penetrated by pathogens. People who have multiple sclerosis, strokes and traumatic brain injuries can have compromised BBBs, meaning that they are vulnerable to all types of infections.

And—I think you were probably waiting for this—inflammatory diseases like diabetes and heart disease, inflammation-causing obesity and yes, Alzheimer's, also weaken the BBB.

Greek Mountain Tea, along with a small number of other botanicals, including rosemary, ashwagandha and quercetin (a potent compound found in onions and garlic) can cross the BBB and all of them actually help reduce inflammation in the brain once they arrive.

GMT's positive effects on the brain begin with its ability to cross the BBB and to increase blood flow to the brain.

The British study on Alzheimer's mentioned in the last chapter had some other interesting findings about brain function not specifically related to dementia or AD.

## Banish test anxiety

Have you ever had test anxiety? It could be the history test in 11th grade or your driver's license exam. You know the feeling: tightness in the belly and maybe in the chest, jitters, maybe a bit of nausea and scattered thoughts.

GMT was shown to relieve those symptoms and help subjects focus clearly and calmly on the task at hand. Better yet, those same individuals first took the test without any assistance from botanicals or prescription drugs and on their second try, with the help of a single dose of GMT, they improved their scores dramatically.

Even though most of us adults don't take exams daily, we are tested on a daily basis, whether we are aware of it or not. Being able to concentrate calmly and put focused attention on your job or your driving, or following a recipe is a most welcome gift.

The human subjects in this British study:

▲ Improved test scores

▲ Improved focus and concentration

▲ Improved scores on high-pressure, rapid-fire visual challenges

▲ Relieved ADHD

▲ Created a sense of calm alertness

▲ Relieved stress and anxiety

After this month-long trial, the results were nothing short of impressive.

The researchers measured responses on a timeline that showed significant improvement in the accuracy of attention, the speed of attention, the working memory to recall words or numbers, how fast they could perform these tasks, how accurate their recall was and their capacity for executive function (performing multiple tasks simultaneously) compared to those given a placebo or ginkgo.

## Brain plasticity

Probably even more significant was the finding that those in the Greek Mountain Tea group also showed improved oxygenated red blood cells in the prefrontal cortex, a part of the brain that governs impulse control, learning, and working memory.

It's more exciting to me that GMT also improved brain plasticity.

A little diversion here: Scientists once thought that we were born with a specific number of brain cells and that number would not change throughout our lives.

Just in the last couple of decades, they discovered this was a deeply false assumption. In fact, we now know that brain cells regenerate throughout our lifetimes. They have the ability to rewire the neural pathways (remember, the brain electrical system) if they are damaged by aging, a stroke or even a head injury.

The confirmation that GMT can assist in this process is tremendously exciting.

## Depression and anxiety

Anxiety and depression are usually the results of faulty brain chemistry. Serotonin and dopamine are chemical messengers (also called neurotransmitters) that govern a broad range of brain signals like pleasurable sensations, attention span, concentration, cognition, memory, mood, alertness and much more.

A third element in depression and anxiety for many people is noradrenaline (sometimes called norepinephrine), which plays dual roles as both a brain messenger and a stress hormone, meaning it has broad effects throughout the entire body.

A German study confirmed that GMT has balancing effects on all three neurotransmitters, acting as a powerful way to address anxiety and depression.

What's more, GMT falls into a new category of substances that treat depression and anxiety called triple monoamine reuptake inhibitors (TRIs). They work precisely on serotonin, dopamine and noradrenaline.

These TRIs are a new generation antidepressant that help overcome the deficiencies in these three brain chemicals, rebalancing them more effectively than previous generations with the serious side effects.

Of course, Greek Mountain Tea is a completely natural substance long known to be effective without side effects, unlike its fellow TRIs like fluoxetine (Prozac).

## ADHD (attention deficit/hyperactivity disorder)

Most of us are familiar with this spectrum of neurodevelopmental disorders of childhood that is becoming distressingly common. These disorders, range from difficulty concentrating to inability to speak and interact to uncontrolled impulses.

ADHD affects about 6 million children and teenagers in the US and, while it likely will dissipate with age, it can affect adults and delay adult brain development as well.

A joint study from Loma Linda University in California, and Korean researchers, concludes that the abundant phenolic compounds in GMT is a safe and effective treatment for ADHD. It works naturally to help rebalance those brain chemicals—serotonin, dopamine and norepinephrine—that can cause depression and anxiety.

The "safe" part of this study is important, since there are stimulant drugs like Adderall, Ritalin, Vyvance, Straterra and Concerta that address ADHD in children and in adults, but they all can have unpleasant side effects like insomnia, loss of appetite, irritability, headaches and more.

GMT to the rescue, again! While the research shows it can be very effective in controlling ADHD, it has no side effects and is safe even for children.

## What's the GMT magic for brain health?

Researchers credit volatile organic compounds, antioxidants and anti-inflammatories in GMT that help calm down misfiring neurons and brain chemicals, promoting optimal brain health.

Some researchers theorize that a strong concentration of acteoside, a polyphenol compound also known as verbascoside, in GMT may be the trigger for restoring brain health and help in the production of GABA (gamma aminobutyric acid), another neurotransmitter that helps elevate mood and a sense of well-being.

Apigenin, another mind-calming flavonoid found in GMT, is a well-researched botanical for reducing anxiety, relaxing muscles and promoting healthy sleep.

### WHAT YOU NEED TO KNOW . . .

In addition of Greek Mountain Tea's memory-enhancing benefits, it can have significant, sometimes profound benefits for general brain health, including:

▲ Overcoming depression and anxiety

▲ Improving focus, concentration and executive skills

▲ Improving test scores and performance

▲ Overcoming ADHD

Not only are these benefits significant, they are achieved naturally through a wide range of complex polyphenols and related compounds that offer natural solutions without side effects found in most drugs.

CHAPTER 6

# GMT's Other Benefits

When I first started studying Greek Mountain Tea, its power against degenerative brain diseases like Alzheimer's deeply impressed me. But when I took another look at its other healing abilities on so many levels, it blew my mind!

Those Greek shepherds have taken advantage of GMT's life-giving properties for millennia. The unassuming scrubby shrub contains healing riches previously unknown to the Western world. Now science has confirmed all of those traditional uses and the healing powers of the *Sideritis scardica* plant. I feel like it's a great honor to be able to share this natural wealth with the world.

As you might imagine from the earlier chapters of this book, GMT's polyphenol abundance is the source of its antioxidant and anti-inflammatory powers and are at the heart of their healing influence over virtually every system of the human body

As you already know, oxidative stress and out-of-control inflammation are primary causes of virtually all chronic diseases, so GMT's antioxidant and anti-inflammatory properties put it high on the list of botanicals to be considered for prevention and treatment of all of these diseases.

## Relieve joint pain, increase stamina

GMT's anti-inflammatory actions are key to the way it supports physical resilience and relieves muscle and joint pain. Shepherding is hard work, so this tea was (and still is) a favorite in the Mediterranean with people who have physically demanding jobs, as well as those working in less strenuous, but still potentially draining and stressful office work.

The energizing aspects of GMT make it an excellent herbal adaptogen, promoting physical stamina without causing jitteriness. It is not caffeinated, and unlike green tea, Greek Mountain Tea has been traditionally recommended in cases of anemia and doesn't deplete iron levels. That may be one of the reasons why the plant was also commonly known as "ironwort"—simply another way of saying "iron plant."

GMT has traditionally been used to aid digestion, strengthen the immune system and suppress common colds, flu and other viruses, allergies, shortness of breath, sinus congestion, even pain and anxiety. Traditionally, GMT has been used to treat urinary tract infections and other microbial attacks.

GMT contains a treasure trove of beneficial polyphenols and other nutrients that can re-energize your mind and body in multiple ways. Its high levels of antioxidants and essential oils, flavonoids, iron and other phytonutrients give it near universal healing powers.

There are *many* reasons to add GMT into a daily regimen.

## Digestive health

Extracts of GMT protect the gastrointestinal system from harm and reduce inflammation. Serbian research shows that GMT is as effective as the now-banned Zantac in preventing inflammation in the gastrointestinal system, especially heartburn. Zantac was banned in 2020 because it was found to cause cancer. As I've noted before, GMT has these impressive effects with no side effects.

GMT also promotes healthy gut bacteria, making it a valuable herbal for assisting in nutrient absorption and keeping your digestive system running smoothly.

Interestingly, the very act of preserving healthy probiotics in the body also helps the polyphenols from Greek Mountain Tea work most effectively. I think that's a good illustration of how there's no separate working system in the body—they're all interconnected, and the way they operate with nutrients is incredibly complex.

Phenolic compounds in GMT have been shown to help the liver efficiently detoxify while also protecting its healthy cells. It activates AMP protein kinase in liver cells, which plays a starring role in how the body unlocks energy from calories, releases hormones and regulates blood sugar levels and metabolism.

In fact, this same Serbian study showed that Greek Mountain Tea reduced blood fats and fasting glucose levels and increased the activity of key antioxidant enzymes. So, aside from general liver function, this botanical could protect against heart disease, type 2 diabetes and weight gain.

## Cancer

Like so many botanicals that have a long history of daily use in their cultures, GMT is a powerful antioxidant and stops free radical damage at a cellular level. In fact, research finds that it is as strong as green tea, even though it contains different compounds and works through different pathways.

That means that GMT has the potential to protect you down to a cellular level from the wear and tear that can spark the beginnings of tumor formations and help you live a longer, healthier life.

GMT provides a compound called acteoside, which promotes a variety of healthy responses in the body. This compound on its own, and various extracts of botanicals that contain it, have been found to inhibit a wide range of cancer types, including prostate, brain and melanoma cancers.

The phenolic compounds in GMT prevent potential cancer development without harming beneficial immune cells. In fact, while GMT is a powerful antioxidant that protects healthy cells, it appears to induce oxidative stress in tumor cells, and ultimately stops them.

## Osteoporosis

Greek research confirms that GMT added to the drinking water of female lab animals who had their ovaries removed, mimicking the hormone profile of post-menopausal women, resulted in impressively increased bone mineral density in just six months.

This is important because more than half of all American women over 50 have some degree of bone loss and about one-third have osteoporosis.

## Finally . . .

In my many years of traveling around the world and researching life-enhancing nutrients, I believe that as an overall tonic for longevity and optimal health, GMT is one of the truly most effective and broad ranging botanicals I've encountered. I urge you to give it a try and add this wonder of the Mediterranean to your daily regimen today.

---

### WHAT YOU NEED TO KNOW . . .

Greek Mountain Tea is traditionally used for a wide range of diseases and illnesses, including:

- ▲ Prevent and treat various types of cancer
- ▲ Relieve gastrointestinal disorders
- ▲ Strengthen the immune system
- ▲ Suppress viral infections including colds, flu and viruses
- ▲ Relieve allergies and sinus infections
- ▲ Reduce shortness of breath
- ▲ Relieve joint pain
- ▲ Protect against osteoporosis

## CHAPTER 7

# Add in Bacopa...

*Bacopa monnieri* has long been used in Ayurvedic medicine to improve brain function, combat memory loss and promote longevity.

Also known as water hyssop or Brahmi, Bacopa is a fuzzy-leafed creeping shrub that grows in wetlands over much of the world.

Modern day research confirms Bacopa's value in improving overall brain health, preserving memory, improving accuracy of recollection and working memory, and helping people perform repetitive tasks while under pressure.

Bacopa contains a wealth of the anti-inflammatory saponin compounds bacosides and bacopasides. These compounds have been shown to enhance cognition, learning and memory. They may also inhibit inflammation in the brain, which we know is an underlying cause of most chronic diseases, including Alzheimer's.

A 2013 study from neuroscientists at Pitzer College in California called Bacopa a "neural tonic and memory enhancer" and attributed its effectiveness to its antioxidant properties, its ability to increase blood flow to the brain, to boost brain chemicals that improve brain function, and to reduce beta amyloid plaques, which we know are commonly found in the brains of people with Alzheimer's.

It's also known to increase levels of the neurotransmitter serotonin, the "feel good" hormone that, among other things, improves sleep and relieves depression and anxiety.

Several studies confirm that Bacopa strengthens the speed of attention and enhances overall cognitive abilities as well as relieving symptoms of depression and anxiety in people of any age.

Some research even shows that Bacopa may help generate new and more efficient neural connections in the brain as we age.

At least one study shows that Bacopa is as effective as rivastigmine (brand name: Exelon), a drug approved to improve cognitive ability in Alzheimer's patients. More importantly, Bacopa has been shown to reverse symptoms of mild cognitive impairment to "normalcy."

Exelon can cause several severe side effects, including aggression and convulsions. Reported side effects of Bacopa are mild gastrointestinal distress.

## ADHD relief

While drugs commonly used to treat this disorder have little or no effect in about 30% of children for whom they are prescribed, Bacopa improved focus and behavior.

Bacopa has near miraculous effects on children with ADHD. A pivotal 2014 Indian study found that Bacopa:

▲ Reduced restlessness in 93% of the children

▲ Improved self-control in 89%

▲ Reduced ADHD symptoms in 85%

## Botanicals v Pharmaceuticals (Prescription Drugs)

I need to pause here for a moment to explore the value of botanicals versus pharmaceuticals. Almost all prescription drugs used today are derived from plants, many from medicinal plants used in traditional healing modalities like Ayurveda and Traditional Chinese Medicine (TCM).

For reasons I cannot completely comprehend, modern developers like to take one or two elements of the total plant that they consider the active ingredients and use it to address a specific medical condition.

They are missing the incredible value of the total plant, and all of its dozens, hundreds, or even thousands of elements that combine in their unique ways to make a total medicine that is highly effective with few, if any, side effects.

It's also worth noting here that many botanicals, like Greek Mountain Tea and Bacopa, can work together to have even greater healing power.

Almost without exception, prescription drugs have side effects, some of them serious and even potentially fatal.

The plant medicines we explore in this book have been verified not only to treat and prevent Alzheimer's, cognitive and brain dysfunction, but to address a broad range of diseases.

Nature is far wiser. The plant world, with medicines in their natural forms, are being proven time and time again to be as effective as prescription drugs without side effects, often for a far lower price.

▲ Reduced learning problems in 78%

▲ Reduced impulsivity in 67%

▲ Improved psychiatric problems in 52%

## Bacopa's other benefits

▲ **CANCER:** Bacopa has impressive anticancer benefits, attacking several types of cancer in at least three different ways: by stopping the wild cell growth typical of cancer, by stopping cancerous tumors from building blood supplies that nourish them, and by stopping the spread of cancer (metastasis).

It has been shown to be effective against colon, breast, liver, prostate and neurological cancers.

In their 2020 review, the Indian researchers called Bacopa "an enriched source of alternative drug development in a nontoxic manner."

▲ **DIABETES:** Bacopa's antioxidant properties helped control blood sugar and even protected against some of the side effects of type 2 diabetes, according to a 2009 Indian animal study.

▲ **CHRONIC PAIN:** In a 2013 review of existing studies at the time, researchers in Pakistan confirmed that Bacopa is an important way of addressing chronic pain and the depression that often accompanies long-term pain. It was also shown to be a safe and effective reliever of neuropathic pain with effectiveness similar to that of opioids without the host of negative side effects of these drugs. It's even been shown to relieve the pain of opioid withdrawal. The researchers concluded that bacopa is a candidate for clinical management of chronic pain.

## Combo power

Here's some great news.

The brain power improvement gets even better when Greek Mountain Tea (GMT) and Bacopa are combined.

German clinical research published in 2016 confirmed that in human subjects with mild cognitive impairment, a combination of Bacopa and GMT was shown to increase beta wave activity in the brain, associated with improving memory and focus.

Those taking the GMT-Bacopa combination also scored better in memory, math and attention tests.

Memory loss is often recognized by family members before the person affected is aware of it. The person experiencing memory loss will sometimes be resistant to the idea, so early detection and treatment become even more important.

Since we know that early detection and treatment of Alzheimer's and other forms of cognitive impairment can slow or even stop the cognitive decline, it's essential to get a diagnosis and start treatment as soon as possible once that memory loss is noticed.

## WHAT YOU NEED TO KNOW

*Bacopa monnieri* is a well-documented way of addressing Alzheimer's disease and cognitive dysfunction by improving:

- ▲ Memory
- ▲ Learning ability
- ▲ Levels of serotonin, the "feel-good" brain chemical that combats anxiety and depression
- ▲ Formation of neurons
- ▲ Ability to perform tasks under pressure
- ▲ Cognitive ability in patients with Alzheimer's disease

It also:

- ▲ Reduces beta amyloid plaque indicative of Alzheimer's disease
- ▲ Improves a variety of manifestations of ADHD

Bacopa is also well documented to:

- ▲ Prevent and treat several types of cancer
- ▲ Control blood sugar in people with type 2 diabetes
- ▲ Help manage chronic pain

A combination of Greek Mountain Tea and Bacopa given to people with mild cognitive impairment improved:

- ▲ Memory
- ▲ Recall
- ▲ Learning ability
- ▲ Focus
- ▲ Attention

CHAPTER 8

# The Right Combo

L et's take a look at the perennial question: How do you find the right product?

I get that question a lot and it's most always followed with another question: How do I know this contains the actual botanical I'm looking for?

And then: How do I know it's safe and not laced with toxins?

Those are all excellent questions.

## Greek Mountain Tea

GMT is a unique botanical because virtually all of it is wildcrafted in the mountains of Greece and surrounding countries.

That means quite literally that local people trek into the mountains and hand harvest the leaves and flowers of the *Sideritis scardica*, carry them to their villages and sell them to distributors.

It's a very simple hands-on operation.

What happens next can be anyone's guess. Loose dried leaves and flowers can be adulterated with other substances, some as benign as other teas, but they can also be prey to contamination during storage or processing.

Also, loose tea cannot be standardized and may have a wide range of essential polyphenol content because of variable growing conditions, rainfall and speed of drying.

That's why I prefer tea processed, tested and standardized into capsules for consistent levels of polyphenols. This is the only way I know of to be certain you are getting a clean product that will do what you need it to do.

Look for a product that is lab tested for purity and quality and contains 500 mg of GMT per capsule with a recommended dosage of one or two a day depending on whether you are taking it for preventive purposes or as a treatment, when the higher dose would be advisable.

As I said in earlier chapters, all you need is one or two capsules daily.

The capsules reassure me that I am getting exactly what I want and need every single day. It's much more convenient, especially if you travel often, as I do.

## *Bacopa monnieri*, a/k/a Bacopa

Look for a product that contains at least 450 mg standardized to contain at least 40% bacosides. Like GMT, one a day would be for prevention, but I suggest you take two a day if you are treating an already existing condition.

I believe the best results will come from taking both GMT and bacopa, especially if you are treating an existing condition, like Alzheimer's or even early memory loss.

As always, you know your own body best and you should consider other supplements you might be taking for potential interactions. There are no serious side effects from either GMT or bacopa, but they can cause mild gastrointestinal problems when you first start taking them. That's why it's best to consult your healthcare practitioner for the best results.

If, as is often the case, your healthcare practitioner is not familiar with GMT or bacopa, please copy the next chapter and offer it as documentation of their potential value in preventing and treating a broad range of conditions, especially Alzheimer's disease and cognitive dysfunction.

> Here are two ways that I suggest using Greek Mountain Tea:
> 1. Greek Mountain Tea, 500 mg capsules, 1 or 2 capsules daily.
>    Or
> 2. A combination of Greek Mountain Tea, 450 mg, with Bacopa, 200 mg per capsule, 1 or 2 capsules daily.

## WHAT YOU NEED TO KNOW . . .

After researching GMT and Bacopa, I believe they should be used together since each enhances the healing properties of the other.

The formula I recommend is 450 mg of Greek Mountain Tea and 200 mg of Bacopa taken together once or twice daily.

Always consult your healthcare practitioner before starting these or any other supplements. If your practitioner is not familiar with these botanicals, please copy the next chapter and offer it to them as documentation.

## CHAPTER 9

# Doc to Doc—
# For Healthcare Professionals

*Dear Readers: We all know our doctors and other healthcare professionals are very busy. As excited as you may be about this book and all it offers, it's unlikely you can persuade a medical professional to read the entire book. That's why we have written this information-packed and very concise summary of the book's contents specifically for people with scientific backgrounds. We encourage you to photocopy, scan or photograph the pages in this chapter and distribute them freely to healthcare professionals. You might want to include the reference section so your practitioner can confirm the research mentioned here.*

### Dear Healthcare Professional:

Your patient has given you a copy of this chapter of *Greek Mountain Tea: The Key to Mental Clarity and More* by Terry Lemerond with our blessings and permission. We have given it to the public domain so that the vital information it contains can be distributed freely.

Our goal is to help medical professionals become familiar with the value of Greek Mountain Tea (*Sideritis scardica*) and *Bacopa monnieri* botanicals that have now been scientifically validated to prevent, treat and even reverse Alzheimer's disease and other neurotransmitter dysfunction.

First, let me briefly introduce myself:

I am Alexander Panossian, Ph.D. and Dr.Sci. in bioorganic chemistry, the chemistry of natural and physiologically active compounds. I have been a professor in this discipline since 1991, working in Sweden since 2003 at the Swedish Herbal Institute and as a founder of Phytomed AB in Sweden. I was editor-in-chief of *Phytomedicine,* an international journal of phytotherapy and phytopharmacology from 2014–2017. I have been credited as lead researcher or participant in more than 180 articles published in peer-reviewed journals, and I hold four US patents. My major interest is in natural botanicals and related medicinals.

I understand that doctors are frequently skeptical about natural formulations and, if they haven't conducted their own investigations on a subject, they are inclined to steer their patients away from them, even though these formulations might be life changing. I urge you to spend a few minutes reviewing these few pages. Confirm them for yourself and consider adding them to your treatment options.

## Greek Mountain Tea (*Sideritus scardica*)

For millennia, Greek Mountain Tea (GMT) has been used to combat cognitive dysfunction in the Ayurvedic medicine tradition.

Now, current human trials confirm that GMT administered at the rate of 950 mg/day for 28 days:

▲ Acts as a triple monoamine transmitter reuptake inhibitor

▲ Increases blood flow to the brain, especially to the prefrontal cortex

▲ Improved flow of oxygen to all body tissues, including to the brain

▲ Slows and reverses formation of beta amyloid plaque

▲ Improved overall cognitive performance

▲ Improved ability to remain focused and access working memory

▲ Improved reaction time

▲ Reduced anxiety

▲ Improved mood

These major findings from a collaboration of British and German researchers concluded that the polyphenols ferulic and chlorogenic acid and the flavonoid apigenin are the likely cause of these benefits.

A German review of more than 4,000 studies on healthy elderly human subjects concluded that specific polyphenols, including those found in GMT, cross the blood-brain barrier, significantly improving information processing speed, executive function and neuron function, while reducing inflammation and free radical oxygen damage in the brain.

In addition, a joint German-Norwegian study published in 2016 confirmed the highly enhanced cognitive function of elderly lab animals given GMT and concluded it "might be a potent, well-tolerated option for treating symptoms of cognitive impairment in the elderly…"

"Well-tolerated" is a key concept here. No serious side effects have been attributable to the use of GMT, even when used on a long-term basis as is common among rural people in Greece and surrounding countries.

## *Bacopa monnieri*

Bacopa has also long been used in Ayurvedic medicine to improve brain function, combat memory loss and promote longevity.

Modern day research confirms Bacopa's value in improving overall brain health, preserving memory, improving accuracy of recollection and working memory, and helping people perform repetitive tasks while under pressure.

Bacopa contains a wealth of the anti-inflammatory saponin compounds bacosides and bacopasides. These compounds have been shown to enhance cognition, learning and memory. They may also inhibit inflammation in the brain, which we know is an underlying cause of most chronic diseases, including Alzheimer's.

A 2013 study from neuroscientists at Pitzer College in California called Bacopa a "neural tonic and memory enhancer" and attributed its effectiveness to its antioxidant properties, its ability to increase blood flow to the brain, to boost neurotransmitters that improve brain function, and to reduce beta amyloid plaques commonly found in the brains of people with Alzheimer's.

Several studies confirm that Bacopa strengthens the speed of attention and enhances overall cognitive abilities as well as relieving symptoms of depression and anxiety in people of any age.

Some research even shows that Bacopa may help generate new and more efficient neural connections in aging brains.

Like GMT, no serious side effects have been associated with Bacopa.

## GMT and Bacopa combined

German clinical research published in 2016 confirmed that in human subjects with mild cognitive impairment, a combination of Bacopa and GMT was shown to increase beta wave activity in the brain, associated with improving memory and focus.

Those taking the GMT-Bacopa combination also scored better in memory, math and attention tests, working at least as effectively at rivastigmine, increasing beta power "seen as a positive effect on pointing to a healthier spectrum."

## CONCLUSION

Much of my research has focused on botanicals known as "adaptogens," the multi-taskers of the plant world. In the simplest possible terms, adaptogens, like GMT and Bacopa, are plant medicines that provide the body what it needs to increase resistance, resilience and to survive.

Adaptogens play a similar role defending the body against environmental challenges, including viruses, harmful bacteria, insect-borne diseases, excessive UV rays and environmental challenges as well as the physiological ravages of chronic stress.

I think of adaptogens as complex compounds that work as science expands and evolves to better understand the disease process. Adaptogens have the potential to provide broad plant-based treatments for complex diseases, chronic conditions and syndromes, including Alzheimer's disease and related cognitive dysfunction.

I strongly urge you to consider leading your patients with Alzheimer's or even age-related cognitive decline on a journey with Greek Mountain Tea and Bacopa. I think you and your patients will be pleasantly surprised.

*—Alexander Panossian, Ph.D. and Dr.Sci.*

# References

### Chapter 2: What Gives GMT Its Kick?

Żyżelewicz D, Kulbat-Warycha K et al. Polyphenols and other bioactive compounds of *Sideritis* plants and their potential biological Activity. *Molecules* 2020 Aug; 25(16): 3763.

### Chapter 4: How GMT Treats and Even Reverses Alzheimer's Disease

Wightman L, Jackson P. The acute and chronic cognitive and cerebral blood flow effects of a *Sideritis scardica* (Greek Mountain Tea) extract: a double blind, randomized, placebo controlled, parallel groups study in healthy humans. *Nutrients*. 2018 Jul 24;10(8):955.

Heiner F, Feistal B et al. *Sideritis scardica* extracts inhibit aggregation and toxicity of amyloid-β in *Caenorhabditis elegans* used as a model for Alzheimer's disease. *PeerJ*. 2018 Apr 30;6:e4683.

Ammar A, Trabelsi K et al. The effect of (poly)phenol-rich interventions on cognitive functions and neuroprotective measures in healthy aging adults: A systematic review and meta-analysis. *J. Clin. Med.* 2020:9(3);835.

Knorl R. Extracts of *Sideritis scardica* as triple monoamine reuptake inhibitors. *J Neural Transm (Vienna)*. 2012 Dec;119(12):1477–82.

Hofrichter J, Krohn M et al. Sideritis spp. Extracts enhance memory and learning in Alzheimer's β-Amyloidosis mouse models and aged C57Bl/6 mice. *J Alzheimers Dis*. 2016 May 31;53(3):967–80.

Behrendt I, Schnieder I et al. Effect of an herbal extract on *Sideritis scardica* and B-vitamins on cognitive performance under stress: a pilot study. *Int J Phytomed*. 2016:8(1);95–103.

### Chapter 5: GMT and Brain Function

Kessler A, Villman C et al. GABA(A) receptor modulation by the volatile fractions of *Sideritis* species used as 'Greek' or 'Turkish' mountain tea. *Flavour and Fragrance Journal* 2012;27(4):297–303.

Ahn J, Ahn H et al. Natural product-derived treatments for attention-deficit/hyperactivity disorder: safety, efficacy and therapeutic potential of combination therapy. *Neural Plast.* 2016;2016:1320423.

## Chapter 6: GMT's Other Benefits

Tadic V, Jeremic I et al. Anti-inflammatory, gastroprotective, and cytotoxic effects of *Sideritis scardica* extracts. *Planta Med.* 2012 Mar;78(5):415–27.

Jeremic I, Petricevic S et al. Effects of *Sideritis scardica* extract on glucose tolerance, triglyceride levels and markers of oxidative stress in ovariectomized rats. *Planta Med.* 2019 Apr;85(6):465–72.

Dontas, I, Lelovas P et al. Protective effect of *Sideritis euboea* extract on bone mineral density and strength of ovariectomized rats. *Menopause.* 2011 Aug;18(8): 915–22.

Tomou E-M, Perrea D et al. Mountain tea (Sideritis plants): a potential anti-atherogenic agent? *J Atheroscleroisi Rev Treat.* 2021; Jan–April 12(1): 27–31.

## Chapter 7: Add in Bacopa . . .

Dimpfel W, Biller A. et al. Psychophysiological effects of a combination of *Sideritis* and *Bacopa* extract (memoLoges®) in 32 Subjects suffering from mild cognitive impairment: a double-blind, randomized, placebo-controlled, 2-armed study with parallel design. *Advances in Alzheimer's Disease.* 2016 Sept;5(3);103–25.

Aguiar S, Borowski T. Neuropharmacological review of the nootropic herb *Bacopa monnieri*. *Rejuvenation Res.* 2013 Aug;16(4):313–26.

Benson S, Downey L. et al. An acute, double-blind, placebo-controlled crossover study of 320 mg and 640 mg doses of *Bacopa monnieri* (CDRI 08) on multitasking stress reactivity and mood. *Phytother Res.* 2014 Apr;28(4):551–59.

Calabrese C, Gregory W et al. Effects of a standardized *Bacopa monnieri* extract on cognitive performance, anxiety, and depression in the elderly: a randomized, double-blind, placebo-controlled trial. *Altern Complement Med.* 2008 Jul;14(6):707–13.

Ghosh S, Khanam R et al. The evolving roles of *Bacopa monnieri* as potential anti-cancer agent: a review. *Nutr Cancer.* 2021;73(11-12):2166–76.

Kapoor R, Sirivastava S et al. *Bacopa monnieri* modulates antioxidant responses in brain and kidney of diabetic rats. *Environ Toxicol Pharmacol.* 2009 Jan;27(1): 62–69.

# Index

**A**

acteoside, 32, 38
AD. *See* Alzheimer's disease (AD)
adaptogens, 36, 55
ADHD (attention deficit/hyperactivity disorder), 12, 27, 29, 31–32, 33, 42, 44, 46
aging, 3, 8, 12, 18
allergies, 36, 39
Alzheimer's disease (AD), 2–3, 5, 6, 12, 13–25, 28, 29, 41, 42, 43, 45, 46, 48, 51, 54, 55
AMP protein kinase, 37
antidepressants, 2, 6, 22, 31
anti-inflammatories, 5, 8, 9, 11, 12, 32, 35, 36, 41, 54
antimicrobials, 2, 11, 36
antioxidants, 3–4, 7–9, 12, 32, 35, 36, 37, 41, 54
anxiety, 2, 12, 21, 22, 23, 25, 27, 29, 31, 32, 33, 36, 42, 46, 53, 54
  *See also* test anxiety
apigenin, 9, 33, 53
ARCD (age-related cognitive decline), 18
ashwagandha, 28
attention. *See* focus

**B**

*Bacopa monnieri*, 41–42, 44–46, 48–49, 54–55
  dosage, 49
  Greek Mountain Tea (GMT) and, 25, 43, 46, 48–49, 55
bacopasides, 41, 54
bacosides, 41, 54
beta amyloid plaque, 15, 23, 25, 41, 46, 53, 54
blood-brain barrier (BBB), 24, 27–28, 53
blood pressure, 2, 6
blood sugar. *See* glucose
bone density, 2, 6, 10, 38
botanicals, 43, 55
brain, 14, 15–16, 18, 24, 25, 27–33, 41, 45, 54
  beta waves, 45, 55
  blood flow to, 22, 23, 25, 28, 41, 52, 54
  cells (*see* neurons)
  executive function of, 24, 25, 30, 33, 53
  plasticity, 30
  prefrontal cortex, 22, 30, 52
breath, 36, 39

59

## C
caffeic acid, 9
cancer, 12, 37–38, 39, 44, 46
cardiovascular disease, 12
carvacrol, 11
cells
   brain (*see* neurons)
   deterioration of, 3, 8
   immune, 38
   liver, 37
chlorogenic acid, 9, 53
cognition, 15–16, 21, 23–24, 25, 41, 42, 46, 53, 54
colds, 2, 6, 11, 36, 39
concentration. *See* focus

## D
Davis, Patti, 13
dementia, 2, 5, 15, 16, 17
dendrites, 16
depression, 2, 6, 12, 21, 22, 25, 31, 32, 33, 42, 44, 54
diabetes (Type 2), 12, 44, 46
digestion, 2, 6, 12, 36–37, 39
diseases, chronic, 4, 8, 12, 35, 41
dopamine, 31, 32

## E
essential oils, 3, 11, 12, 36

## F
ferulic acid, 53
flavonoids, 3, 7, 33, 36, 53
flu, 2, 6, 11, 36, 39
focus, 22, 24, 25, 29, 33, 41, 42, 45, 46, 53, 54, 55
free radicals, 3, 8, 24, 37, 53

## G
GABA (gamma aminobutyric acid), 32
glucose, 28, 37, 44, 46
Greek Mountain Tea (GMT), 1–3, 5, 6, 7, 21–25, 47–48, 52–53
   *Bacopa monnieri* and, 43, 45, 48, 49, 55
   capsules, 5, 7, 48
   dosage, 48, 49

## H
heartburn, 37
Hippocrates, 1–2

## I
immune system, 2, 28, 36, 39
inflammation, 3, 5, 8, 16, 25, 28, 35, 37, 41, 53, 54
insulin resistance, 2, 6
iron, 36
ironwort. *See* Greek Mountain Tea (GMT)

## J
joints, 2, 6, 36, 39

## K
kaempherol, 9

## L
liver, 37

## M
math tests, 45, 55
MCI (mild cognitive impairment), 16, 42, 45, 46, 55
memory and memory loss, 16, 17, 19, 22, 23, 24, 30, 45, 46, 53, 54, 55
minerals, 10–11, 12
monoterpenes, 11
moods, 22, 32, 53

## N

neural pathways, 16, 25, 30, 42, 54
neurons, 15, 24, 25, 30, 42, 46, 53, 54
neuropathy, 44
neurotransmitters, 31, 32, 42, 54
noradrenaline, 31, 32
norepinephrine. *See* noradrenaline

## O

opioids, 44
ORAC scale, 8, 9
osteoporosis, 38, 39
oxidation, 3
oxidative stress, 4, 5, 35, 38,
oxygen, 3, 52

## P

pain, chronic, 44, 46
phenolic compounds. *See* polyphenols
picture recognition, 22
pinene, 11
pneumonia, 17
polyphenols, 4, 7–9, 12, 23–24, 32, 35, 36, 37, 38, 48, 53
probiotics, 37

## Q

quercetin, 9, 28

## R

reaction time, 23, 53
Reagan, Ronald, 13
rosemary, 28

## S

saponins, 41, 54
serotonin, 31, 32, 42, 46
*Sideritis scardica*. *See* Greek Mountain Tea (GMT)
sinuses, 36, 39
stamina, 36
stress, 24, 25, 29
synergy, 43, 45, 49

## T

tasks, 16, 46
    problem-solving, 16, 24, 29, 45, 55
    repetitive, 25, 41, 54
tau tangles, 16
test anxiety, 29–30
triple monoamine reuptake inhibitors (TRIs), 22, 31, 52
tumors, 38, 44

## U

urinary tract infections, 36

## V

verbascoside. *See* acteoside
viruses, 36, 39
vitamin B1, 24
vitamin B6, 24
vitamin B12, 24

## W

weight loss, 2, 6
word recall, 30, 46
wound healing, 2, 6, 11

# About the Author

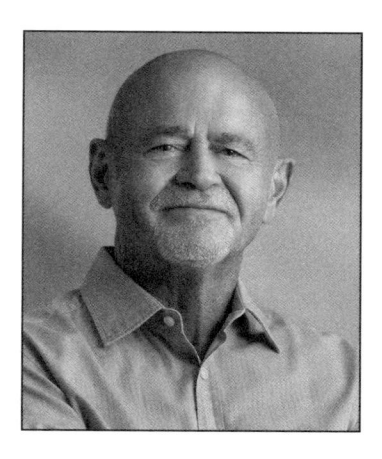

**Terry Lemerond** is a natural health expert with over 50 years of experience. He has owned health food stores, founded dietary supplement companies and formulated over 400 products.

A much sought-after speaker and accomplished author, Terry shares his wealth of experience and knowledge in health and nutrition through social media, newsletters, podcasts, webinars, and personal speaking engagements. His books include *Seven Keys to Vibrant Health* and the sequel, *Seven Keys to Unlimited Personal Achievement,* and his newest publication, *50+ Natural Health Secrets Proven to Change Your Life.* His continual dedication, energy, and zeal are part of his on-going mission—to improve the health of America.

# KNOWLEDGE IS POWER,
## ESPECIALLY FOR YOUR HEALTH!

Are you in search of a reliable, science-based resource for all your health and nutrition questions? Terry Talks Nutrition has you covered.

Connect with Terry to increase your knowledge on a wide variety of topics, including immunity, pain, curcumin and cancer, diabetes, and so much more!

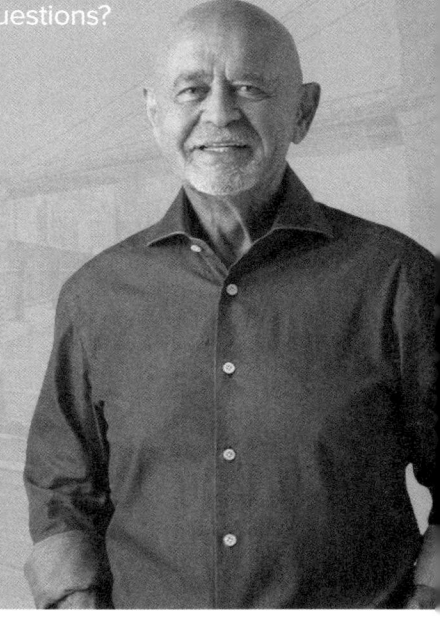

## READ
Visit TerryTalksNutrition.com for today's latest and greatest health and nutrition information.

## LISTEN
Tune in on Sat. and Sun. 8-9 am (CST) at TerryTalksNutrition.com for a live internet radio show hosted by Terry! You can listen to past shows on the website or on your favorite podcast app.

## ENGAGE
Connect with us on Facebook, where you can engage with other individuals seeking safe and effective ways to improve overall wellness.

## WATCH
Check out our educational YouTube Channel to learn from the world's leading doctors and health experts.

Simply open your smartphone camera. Hold over desired code above for more information.

Get answers to all of your health questions at **TERRYTALKSNUTRITION.COM**

## WELCOME TO

# ttn publishing

Are you ready to learn how anyone can use natural medicines, safely and effectively, to improve their health? You'll love TTN Publishing, my newest endeavor to bring you cutting edge research on powerful, health-supporting botanicals. I've coauthored numerous books with top alternative doctors from around the world to help you learn all you can about taking your health into your own hands. These educational books, supported by powerful scientific research, contain all the information you need to live a life of vibrant health.

In Good Health,
Terry Lemerond

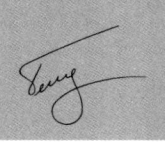

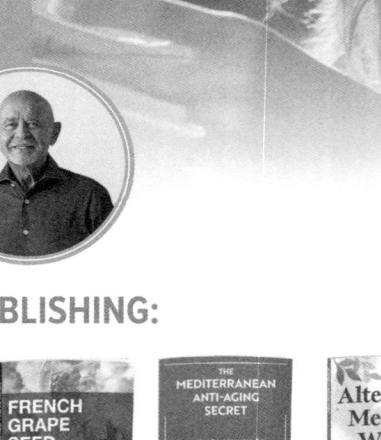

## ADDITIONAL BOOKS BY TTN PUBLISHING:

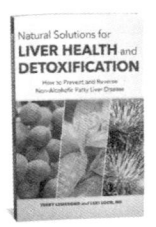

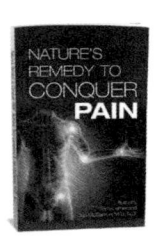

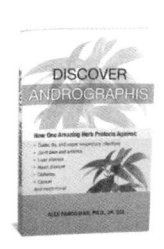

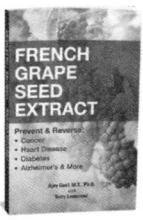

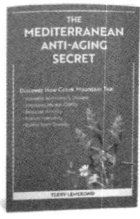

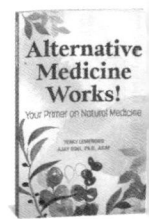

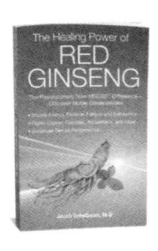

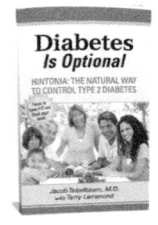

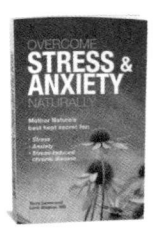

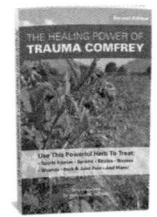

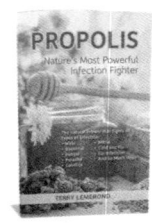

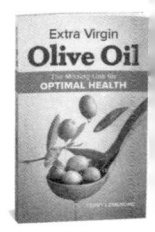

- Natural Solutions for LIVER HEALTH and DETOXIFICATION
- NATURE'S REMEDY TO CONQUER PAIN
- DISCOVER ANDROGRAPHIS
- FRENCH GRAPE SEED EXTRACT
- THE MEDITERRANEAN ANTI-AGING SECRET
- Alternative Medicine Works!
- The Healing Power of RED GINSENG
- Diabetes Is Optional
- OVERCOME STRESS & ANXIETY NATURALLY
- THE HEALING POWER of TRAUMA COMFREY
- PROPOLIS Nature's Most Powerful Infection Fighter
- Extra Virgin Olive Oil

Get a copy for yourself and gift them to the people you care about!

©2024_01_EP187